THE LITTLE
BOOK OF WRINKLES

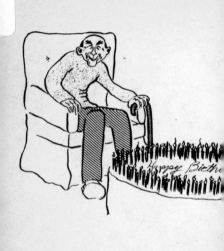

THE LITTLE
BOOK OF WRINKLES

Compiled &

Annotated by

EVELYN STEINBERG &

MARILYN WILLIAMS

SERIES EDITOR
STEPHEN OSBORNE
A LITTLE RED BOOK
ARSENAL PULP PRESS

A Little Red Book

THE LITTLE BOOK OF WRINKLES
TEXT AND ILLUSTRATIONS
COPYRIGHT © 1993
BY EVELYN STEINBERG &
MARILYN WILLIAMS
All rights reserved.
ISBN 0-88978-264-4
CIP DATA: *see page 6*

LITTLE RED BOOKS
are published by
ARSENAL PULP PRESS
1062 HOMER STREET #100
VANCOUVER BC V6B 2W9
COVER DESIGN: *Kelly Brooks*
ILLUSTRATIONS: *Eve Corbel*
TYPESETTING: *Vancouver Desktop*
PRINTING: *Webcom*
PRINTED AND BOUND IN CANADA

TABLE OF CONTENTS

CANADIAN CATALOGUING
IN PUBLICATION DATA

Main entry under title:
The Little book of wrinkles
   (A Little red book)
   ISBN 0-88978-264-4

   1. Aging—Quotations, maxims, etc.
2. Aging—Humour. 3. Quotations, En-
glish. I. Steinberg, Evelyn, 1944-
II. Williams, Marilyn, 1935-   III. Series.
PN6084.A35L58 1993   305.26'0207
C93-091391-4

If you live long enough, my grand-
mother once said, you get to see everything twice. I don't know if she
meant this for better or for worse, but
I was moved to inscribe her words in
my diary twenty-five years ago, and
recall them now with the pleasing
melancholy that attends the making
of small memorials. Memorials of
course are another way of marking
time—surely one of our oldest cultural practices. Time in its recurring
mode we mark with calendars and
almanacs of seasons and days; time in
its sweeping-all-before-it mode we

can only note in passing, with verse and epigram, adage and remark—and memorials such as the present volume, which, while teasing us to gaze upon eternity, dares us to stare into oblivion.

The following pages represent the careful gleaning of some 2,600 years of mediation, speculation and study. Doubtless there remains still more to be found, but as we have no more pages to fill, we need concern ourselves no longer with searching them out. The compilers have earned their rest; now the publishers will earn theirs. Herein you will find much that instructs and more that delights: all of art's ancient purposes fulfilled.

Where approriate, we have appended dates and other notes that will provide useful to students and, we hope, challenging to wordsmiths. Time in its form of kinesis, we are reminded, is always running out.

—*S. Osborne*

THE QUOTATIONS

POSSIBLY ONE OF LIFE'S
GREATEST COMFORTS

I used to dread getting older because I thought I would not be able to do all the things I wanted to do, but now that I'm older I find that I don't want to do them.

— Nancy, Lady Astor, first woman to sit in the British House of Commons

ENTAILING ONE OF LIFE'S
GREATEST REWARDS

Ah well, perhaps one has to be very old before one learns how to be amused rather than shocked.

— Pearl S. Buck, American writer

NOT TO MENTION THE
BENEVOLENT
SIDE EFFECTS

By the time the average man is old enough to gratify his tastes, he hasn't any.
— Bob Edwards, Canadian publisher & writer, *Calgary Eye Opener*, 1915

TRULY A
GREAT NOTION

Old folks are the nation.
— Toni Cade Bambera, writer, pioneer in black women's literature

SOMETHING TO
LOOK
FORWARD TO, THEN

It must be pleasant to reach that

age when one can go to the lavatory
without explanation.
— Enid Bagnold, novelist, *The Chinese
Prime Minister*, 1964

ALL YOU REALLY
NEED
TO KNOW, REALLY

The secret of staying young is to
live honestly, eat slowly, and lie
about your age.
— Lucille Ball, American comedienne

SOMETHING,
THOUGH,
TO PRAY FOR

Few women, I fear, have had such
reason as I have to think the long
sad years of youth were worth liv-

ing for the sake of middle age.
— George Eliot, English novelist

BUT RALPH,
WHATEVER
HAPPENED TO
NATURAL CAUSES?

Nature abhors the old, and old age seems the only disease; all others run into this one.
— Ralph Waldo Emerson,
American poet & essayist

WHAT WE NEED TO
HEAR MORE OF

Old age, believe me, is a good and pleasant thing. It is true you are gently shouldered off the stage, but then you are given such a comfort-

able front stall as spectator.
— Jane (Ellen) Harrison,
English writer

A SUBJECT ALWAYS
RIPE FOR
METAPHORICAL OVERKILL

To know how to grow old is the masterwork of wisdom, and one of the most difficult chapters in the great art of living.
— Henri-Frédérick Amiel, Swiss philosopher and writer, *Journal Intime*, 1883

ON WHEN ONE OUGHT TO
BE PREPARING ONESELF

Preparing for the worst is an activity I have taken up since I turned thirty-five, and the worst actually began to happen.

— Delia Ephron, American writer

SURE, IN A PERFECT WORLD

In youth we learn; in age we understand.

— Marie Ebner von Eschenbach, Austrian writer

IT WOULDN'T BE COMPLETE, OF COURSE, WITHOUT THE IRONY

Youth, which is forgiven everything, forgives itself nothing: age, which forgives itself anything, is forgiven nothing.

— George Bernard Shaw

EFFECT OF GREAT WEALTH
ON THE VICISSITUDES OF AGE

Here I must say, in my eighty-sixth year, I do not feel greatly different from when I was eighty-five.

> — William Maxwell Aitken (Lord Beaverbrook), Canadian-British politician, newspaper proprietor

AND SO LITTLE TO
GRIPE ABOUT, TOO

I once had youth, and I now have success.

> — William Maxwell Aitken (Lord Beaverbrook), *The Three Keys to Success*, 1956

SOMETIMES IT HELPS
TO BE A MOVIE STAR

If you survive long enough, you're revered—rather like an old building.

— Katharine Hepburn, American actress

A CONUNDRUM FOR
THE CURIOUS

Nothing seems so tragic to one who is old as the death of one who is young, and this alone proves that life is a good thing.

— Zöe Akins, American writer

TO EVERY
SILVER LINING

One of the chief pleasures of middle age is looking back at the people you didn't marry.

— Anonymous

THERE'S ALWAYS A SOMETHING OR OTHER

Don't worry about avoiding temptation. As you get older, it will avoid you.

— Equally anonymous

YES, BUT ONLY FOR ONE NIGHT, PLEASE

Backward, turn backward, O
Time, in your flight,
Make me a child again just
*   for tonight.*

— Elizabeth Akers Allen,
"Rock Me To Sleep," 1860

ON WHAT TO
EXPECT FROM
HINDSIGHT

The only thing I regret about my life is the length of it. If I had to live my life again I'd make all the same mistakes—only sooner.

— Tallulah Bankhead, actress

SOME METAPHORS
INVITE EXTENSION

It is sad to grow old but nice to ripen.

— Brigitte Bardot, French actress

USUALLY AT THE
RISK OF THE
METAPHOR-MAKER

It is not all bad, this getting old,

this ripening. After the fruit has got its growth it should juice up and mellow. God forbid I should live long enough to ferment and rot and fall to the ground in a squash.

— Emily Carr, Canadian painter, writer

LITTLE-KNOWN
BENEFIT OF
GROWING OLD

Old people shouldn't eat health foods. They need all the preservatives they can get.

— Anonymous

SOME THINGS
REMAIN ETERNAL

Young men think old men are fools; but old men know young

men are fools.

— George Chapman, English dramatist,
All Fools, 1605

AND OTHERS ARE
MERELY PLAGIARISM

Old fellers always think young ones fools, but young fellers sometimes know old ones is fools.

— Thomas Chandler Haliburton (a.k.a. Sam Slick), Canadian humourist

UNMISTAKEABLE SIGN
OF MIDDLE AGE

My youth is escaping without giving me anything it owes me.

— Ivy Compton-Burnett, English writer,
A Heritage and Its History, 1959

NEARBY THE INEFFABLE
TRUTH ALWAYS LURKING

There is no bar mitzvah for menopause.

— Pauline Bart

WHAT MENOPAUSE IS
ANYTHING BUT

Calm and poise do not simply happen to the post-menopausal woman: she has to fight for them. When the fight is over, her altered state might look to a younger woman like exhaustion, when it is really anything but. I wouldn't have missed it for the world.

— Germaine Greer, American writer

THE QUANTUM MECHANICS
OF AGING

We grow old by moments and not by years.

— Beverley Baxter, Canadian journalist, *Strange Street*, 1935

THE RELATIVISTIC
VIEW

Just remember, once you're over the hill, you begin to pick up speed.

— Anonymous

DEFINITION OF
A MOMENT
OF AGING

I always wanted to be old, I wanted to say / I haven't read that for fifteen years.

— John Berryman, poet, Poem No. 264,
His Toy, His Dream, His Rest, 1968

ON THE SEEMLY

AND

THE UNSEEMLY

'You are old, Father William,'
the young man said,
'And your hair has become very
white;
And yet you incessantly stand on
your head—
Do you think at your age, it is
right?'

— Lewis Carroll,
Alice's Adventures in Wonderland

SIGNS OF
WHAT'S AHEAD

Whenever a man's friends begin to compliment him about looking young, he may be sure that they think he is growing old.

— Washington Irving, American writer,
Bracebridge Hall, 1822

WELL, IT COULD BE OPENING
THOSE INFURIATING
RUSSIAN DOLLS,
WE SUPPOSE,
OR PEELING ONIONS,
OR WHATHAVEYOU

Perhaps middle age is, or should be, a period of shedding shells; the shell of ambition, the shell of material accumulations and possessions,

the shell of the ego.
— Anne Morrow Lindbergh,
American writer

**BUT WHEN HAVE THEY
BOTHERED COMING AFTER
ANYONE AT ALL?**
Do knights on white chargers ever
bother coming after women whose
sagging chin folds are showing?
— Maggie Scarf, American writer,
Unfinished Business, 1980

**ON WHAT HAPPENS
WHEN THE DEVIL
TAKES OVER**
From thirty-five to forty-five,
women are old; but at forty-five,
the devil takes over and they

become beautiful, splendid, maternal, proud. The acidities are gone and in their place reigns calm. These women are worth going out to find and because of them some men never grow old. When I see them my mouth waters.

— Jean-Bapiste Troisgros

PROOF THAT NOT ENOUGH
EDITORS GROW OLD
IN HARNESS

It is hard to convince editors that people of or past forty are not senile, and might even have problems, emotions, and—mirabile dictu—romances, licit and illicit.

— Faith Baldwin,
American writer

THE REWARDS
ARE FEW
BUT GRATIFYING

The lovely thing about being forty is that you can appreciate twenty-five year-old men more.

> — Colleen McCullough,
> Australian novelist

ON BEING TRAPPED
COMING
OR GOING

Love? For whom? An old man? How horrible. A young man? How shameful.

> — Coco Chanel, French
> fashion designer

NOT TO PUT TOO FINE
A POINT ON IT

Every man over forty is a scoundrel.

— George Bernard Shaw

ANCIENT TRUTHS ON
PREMATURE AGING

Envy and wrath shorten the life, and carefulness bringeth age before the time.

— The Bible, Ecclesiasticus 30:24

NOT THAT MUCH DIFFERENT
FROM THE YOUNGER
VARIETY, WHEN YOU
THINK ABOUT IT

Old men are like that, you know. It makes them feel important to think

they are in love with somebody.
— Willa Cather, American writer,
My Antonia, 1915

MORE MIXED AND

ANCIENT

METAPHORS

Old age: the crown of life, our
play's last act.
— Marcus Tullius Cicero, Roman
statesman, *De Senectute*

MEANWHILE THE SEARCH

FOR CANADIAN

METAPHORS

ONGOETH

While there's snow on the roof, it
doesn't mean the fire has gone out

in the furnace.
— John G. Diefenbaker,
Canadian politician

ONE OF LIFE'S
LITTLE IRONIES

People who are old enough to know better often wish they were young enough not to.
— Bob Edwards, Canadian publisher & writer, *Calgary Eye Opener*, 1922

SIDE EFFECTS OF JOINING
IN THE RAT RACE

By the time we've made it, we've had it.

— Anonymous

AND THEN SENDS THEM OFF
TO WAR ANYWAY

Young men's minds are always changeable, but when an old man is concerned in a matter, he looks both before and after.

— Homer, c. 700 B.C., *The Iliad*

THE DREAM OF LIFE: A
MERCANTILE VIEW

Youth is the time of getting, middle age of improving, and old age of spending.

— Anne Bradstreet, English poet, *Meditations Divine and Moral*, 1664

HOW TO KNOW THE DANCER
FROM THE DANCE

It is not that I belong to the past but

that the past belongs to me.
— Mary Antin, American writer

WHAT MIGHT BE
THE WORST OF IT

What is the worst of woes that
wait on age?
What stamps the wrinkle deeper
on the brow?
To view each loved one blotted
from life's page,
And be alone on earth, as I am
now.
— Lord Byron, English poet, "Childe
Harold's Pilgramage," 1812

AND WHAT MIGHT BE THE BEST

As a white candle
In a holy place,

So is the beauty
of an aged face.

—Joseph Campbell,
"The Old Woman"

ANCIENT FEARS
REVISTED

Cast me not off in the time of old age; forsake me not when my strength faileth.

— The Bible, Psalms 71:9

JUST ANOTHER OF THOSE
NEVER-TO-BE-
SUBSTANTIATED SIMILES?

Being an old maid is like death by drowning, a really delightful sensation after you cease to struggle.

— Edna Ferber, American novelist

A SUBJECT TO INVOKE
INCOHERENCE IN THE MOST
SURPRISING OF PEOPLE

There is a denial of the personhood of people over sixty-five. What values emerge if you don't measure everything in terms of youth? What is that human being like?

— Betty Friedan, American writer

ON SILLINESS AND
ACTING
YOUR AGE

I'm not interested in age. People who tell their ages are silly. You're as young as you feel.

— Elizabeth Arden, Canadian-American
businesswoman

WHAT TO EXPECT WHEN
THE METAPHORS DRY UP

After seventy, one's reason tells one that the anticipation of many more years of life is not justifiable; one should count every year after one's seventieth as "velvet."

— Lewellys F. Barker, Canadian physician, *Time and the Physician*, 1942

UNPLEASANT TRUTHS
DEPT: THE
CALIFORNIA EFFECT

You know, when I first went into the movies, Lionel Barrymore played my grandfather. Later he played my father and finally he played my husband. If he had lived, I'm sure I would have played his mother. That's the way it is in Hollywood. The men get younger and the women get older.

— Lillian Gish, American actress

INTIMATIONS OF
A VERY
SATISFYING KIND

The old woman I shall become will be quite different from the woman I am now. Another I is beginning and so far I have not had to complain of her.

— George Sand, French writer,
Isadora

WHAT WE KNEW
ONCE TO BE
BENEVOLENT SENESCENCE

Old men are children for the second time.

— Aristophanes, Greek playwright,
Clouds, 423 B.C.

TRUTH BEHIND
THEORIES OF
BENEVOLENT SENESCENCE

Age does not make us childish as they say. / It only finds us true children still.

— Johann Wolfgang von Goethe,
German poet, dramatist, scientist,
Faust, 1832

NOT-SO-BENEVOLENT
IMPLICATIONS OF
SAID SENESCENCE

Wives are young men's mistresses, companions for middle age, and old men's nurses.

— Francis Bacon, English philosopher,
Essays, 1625

AND TRY TO KEEP THE
WHINGING OUT OF IT, TOO

While others may argue about whether the world ends with a bang or a whimper, I just want to make sure mine doesn't end with a whine.

— Barbara Gordon, American TV
producer and writer

ANOTHER SHOT IN
THE BATTLE
FOR THE LAST WORD

The young man who has not wept
is a savage, and the old man who
will not laugh is a fool.

— George Santayana, Spanish
philosopher, poet, novelist

BUT HOW THEN
ARE WE
TO LAMENT
THE WORLD OF
CONSUMERIST IMAGERY?

One searches the magazines in vain
for women past their first youth.
The middle-aged face apparently
sells neither perfume nor floor
wax. The role of the mature

woman in the media is almost en-
tirely negative.

> — Janet (Dorothea) Harris,
> American writer,
> *The Prime of Ms. America*, 1975

ON ATTAINING
THE FREEDOM
OF ANONYMITY.

All one's life as a young woman one
is on show, a focus of attention,
people notice you. You set yourself
up to be noticed and admired. And
then, not expecting it, you become
middle-aged and anonymous. No
one notices you. You achieve a
wonderful freedom. It is a positive
thing. You can move about unno-

ticed and invisible.
> — Doris Lessing, English novelist,
> playwright

ONLY TAKE YOUR
METAPHORS
AS FAR AS YOU DARE

Your skins are taut.
Your faces smooth
like fresh plums.
My skin is wrinkled.
My brow furrowed
like a prune.
Prunes are sweeter.
> — Natasha Josephowitz, Professor of
> Management, lecturer,
> *Is This Where I Was Going?*

THOSE PRE-EXISTENTIALIST EXISTENTIALISTS COULD BE A PRETTY DREARY BUNCH IN THEIR MIDDLE AGE

Youth is a blunder; manhood a struggle; old age a regret.

— Benjamin Disraeli, English statesman, novelist, *Coningsby*, 1844

TO TAKE A RATHER PLATITUDINOUS APPROACH

By the time we hit fifty, we have learned our hardest lessons. We have found out that only a few things are really important. We have learned to take life seriously, but never ourselves.

— Marie Dressler, actress, *My Own Story*, 1934

MORE ON
RELATIVITY

You know, I've made an interesting discovery. You don't change when you grow old. You remain the same. But everything else changes. Your home. Your friends. Your city. The things you are used to just disappear, one by one. And you are left alone.

— Gregory Clark, Canadian journalist

RELIEVED BY
THE SIMPLE LYRIC

Then welcome Age and fear not
*   sorrow;*
Today's no better than tomorrow.

— Alice Corbin, American poet,

Two Voices

Aging people should know that their lives are not mounting and unfolding but that an inexorable inner process forces the contradiction of life. For a young person it is almost a sin—and certainly a danger—to be too much occupied with himself; but for the aging person it is a duty and a necessity to give serious attention to himself.

— Carl Gustav Jung,
Swiss psychiatrist, *Modern Man
in Search of a Soul*, 1933

SURELY WE'VE HEARD
THIS ONE BEFORE

Of late I have searched diligently to discover the advantage of age, and there is, I have concluded, only one. It is that lovely young women treat your approaches with understanding rather than with disdain.

— John Kenneth Galbraith,
Canadian-American economist, author

MORE PROOF THAT NOT ALL
ONE-LINERS AGE AS
WELL AS THEIR OWNERS

You can't help getting older but you don't have to get old.

— George Burns,
American comedian

WHAT WE REALLY
LIKE TO DO

Old people like to give good advice, as solace for no longer being able to provide good examples.

— François, Duc de La Rochefoucauld,
French writer, *Reflections*

ONE OF THE LASTING
GREAT COMFORTS

Amidst the infirmities of age, it is a great comfort to old folks that, whatever destruction time works in their memory, they never find it affecting their judgement.

— Thomas McCulloch, church minister,
educator, writer

TRUE, BUT WOULDN'T ONE OF ANY DOZEN EPITHETS DO AS WELL?

When a man drops out at the age of eighty, people can't say he's a quitter.

— W.R. Motherwell, Canadian politician

NOW WHAT HAVE WE ALL SECRETLY SUSPECTED?

Old women snore violently. They are like bodies into which bizarre animals have crept at night; the animals are vicious, bawdy, noisy. How they snore! There is no shame to their snoring. Old women turn into old men.

— Joyce Carol Oates, American writer, in *Mademoiselle*, February 1960

**AND WHAT HAVE WE
SECRETLY DESIRED?**

I'd like to grow very old as slowly
as possible.

— Irene Mayer Selznick,
theatrical producer

**A SIGN, OR A
PERQUISITE?**

That sign of old age, extolling the
past at the expense of the present.

— Sydney Smith, English essayist,
Lady Holland's Memoir, 1855

**ESPECIALLY IF YOU'RE NOT
ALREADY SAVING
UP FOR THE RV**

Education is the best provision for

old age.

— Aristotle, Greek philosopher, *Diogenes Laertius, Lives of Eminent Philosophers*, c. 340 BC.

ON NOT MINDING
NEVER REALLY BEING
ABLE TO STOP WORRYING

Actually, I have only two things to worry about now: afterlife and re-incarnation.

— Gail Parent, American writer, "The End," *Sheila Levine is Dead and Living in New York*, 1972

MORE SALUBRIOUS
SIDE EFFECTS

I am not half as patient with old

women now that I am one.
— Emily Carr, Canadian painter, writer,
Hundreds and Thousands, 1940

REMARKS, OF COURSE,
DO NOT A LITERATURE MAKE
A woman is as good as her knees.
— Mary Quant, English fashion designer

MORE MIXED AND
ANCIENT METAPHOR
*And what's a life?—a weary pil
grimage,
Whose glory in one day doth fill
the stage
With childhood, manhood, and
decrepit age.*
— Francis Quarles, English poet, c. 1635

ON WHAT IS IN WHEN
THE OTHER IS OUT

A good old man, sir; he will be talking: as they say, When the age is in, the wit is out.

— William Shakespeare,
Much Ado About Nothing

THE RHETORICAL QUESTION
FOREVER WAITING TO BE ASKED

Who would return to the youth he is forever pretending to regret?

— Agnes Repplier, American writer,
social critic,
Books and Men, 1888

REMEMBER WHEN, OR:
THE ANGST, THE ANGST!

It's so horrible to be—oh God—

thirty. . . . . Today is a turning point in my life, the beginning of the end. It's pushing forty—and menopause out there waiting to spring—and before you can even turn around you're a senior citizen.

— Muriel Resnick, American playwright,
Any Wednesday, 1963

WHAT TO EXPECT WHEN
MEDIUM-HIGH SERIOUSNESS
BEGINS TO REPLACE A
SENSE OF HUMOUR

Have you ever been out for a late autumn walk in the closing part of the afternoon, and suddenly looked up to realize that the leaves have practically all gone? You had not realized it. And you notice that the sun has set already, the day before you knew it—and with that a cold wind blows across the landscape. That's retirement.

— Stephen Leacock,
Canadian humourist, 1939

MEDITATION ON
REMAINING EXCESSIVELY
IDLE IN ONE'S DOTAGE

*There was an Old Man with a
beard,
Who said: 'It is just as I feared!
Two owls and a hen
Four larks and a wren,
Have all built their nests in my
beard.'*

— Edward Lear, English humourist,
Book of Nonsense, 1846

SURELY YOU COULD AT LEAST
START DEMANDING
MORE FREE DRINKS

Old age is like a plane flying through a storm. Once you are aboard there is nothing you can do. You can't stop the plane, you can't stop the storm, you can't stop time. So one might as well accept it calmly, wisely.

— Golda Meir, Israeli Prime Minister

TO SAY FAREWELL TO
THE SPORTING LIFE,
AND JUST RELAX

There are compensations for growing older. One is the realization that to be sporting isn't at all necessary. It is a great relief to

reach this state of wisdom.
— Cornelia Otis Skinner, American
writer, actress,
Dithers and Jithers, 1937

WHAT TO REMEMBER
UPON FIRST
DOUBTING ONESELF

If, as you grow older, you feel you are also growing stupider, do not worry. This is normal, and usually occurs around the time when your children, now grown, are discovering the opposite—they now see that you aren't nearly as stupid as they had believed when they were teenagers.

— Margaret Laurence,
Canadian novelist

SOME THINGS THAT ONE CAN
DO IN ONE'S DOTAGE

King David and King Solomon
Led merry, merry lives,
With many, many friends
And many, many wives;
But when old age crept over
them—
With many, many qualms,
King Solomon wrote the Proverbs
And King David wrote the
Psalms.
 — James Ball Naylor, *Ancient Authors*

WHAT WE SECRETLY
HOLD
TO BE TRUE

An excellent recipe for longevity is
this: cultivate a minor ailment, and

take very good care of it.
— William Osler,
Canadian physician

ON THE PLACE OF
SELF-INTEREST
IN MEDICAL RESEARCH

I'm interested in geriatrics because
I'm going to be old some day too.
— Robert McClure,
Canadian medical missionary

GOOD NEWS FOR
THE CHRONICALLY
CALM AND HAPPY

He who is of calm and happy nature will hardly feel the pressure of
age, but to him who is of an opposite disposition youth and age are

equally a burden.

> — Plato, *The Republic*

WHERE NON-SEQUITORS
TEND TO
LEAD ONE

Middle-aged rabbits don't have a paunch, do have their own teeth and haven't lost their romantic appeal.

> — Aurelia Poter, American physician

MUSIC THAT FEEDS THE SOUL

You are beautiful and faded,
Like an old opera tune
Played upon a harpsichord.
— Amy Lowell, American poet, "A Lady,"
Sword Blades and Poppy Seeds, 1914

THE RHETORIC OF
THE ONE-LINER

A woman's a woman until the day she dies, but a man's only a man as long as he can.
— Moms Mabley, American entertainer

THE SELF-RIGHTEOUS
ARE FOREVER
WITH US

When you cease to make a contribution you begin to die.
— Eleanor Roosevelt,
American First Lady

MORE WAYS THAN
ONE TO RAGE AGAINST
THE DYING OF THE LIGHT

I refuse to admit I'm more than

fifty-two even if that does make my
sons illegitimate.

— Nancy, Lady Astor, English politician,
first woman to sit in the British House
of Commons

ON TURNING

UNCONTROLLABLE

Time and trouble will tame an ad-
vanced young woman, but an ad-
vanced   old   woman   is
uncontrollable by any earthly
force.

— Dorothy L. Sayers, English writer,
Clouds of Witness, 1956

NO DOUBT ALREADY A

WELL-WORN SAW

Alonso of Aragon was wont to say

in commendation of age, that age appears to be best in four things— old wood best to burn, old wine to drink, old friends to trust, and old authors to read.

— Francis Bacon, English philosopher, *Apothegms*, 1624

TO BE REVIVED EVERY
HUNDRED YEARS OR SO
I love everything that's old: old friends, old manners, old books, old wines.

— Oliver Goldsmith, Irish writer

ENCOURAGING LIGHT
FUTHER UP
THE TUNNEL
Age puzzles me. I thought it was

quite a time. My seventies were interesting and fairly serene, but my eighties are passionate. I grow more intense as I age.

— Florida Scott-Maxwell,
American-Scottish writer,
The Measure of My Days, 1972

WHAT PERSISTS, BUT
THE ETERNAL VERITIES?
When men reach their sixties and retire, they go to pieces. Women go right on cooking.

— Gail Sheehy, American writer

WHERE THE REVELATION
COMES FROM
Since it is the Other within us who is old, it is natural that the revela-

tion of our age should come to us
from outside—from others. We do
not accept it willingly.

— Simone de Beauvoir,
French writer, philosopher,
The Coming of Age, 1972

WHAT EVERY GOOD

QUOTATION BOOK

NEEDS AT

LEAST ONE OF

If anything is a surprise then there
is not much difference between
older and younger because the only
thing that does make anybody
older is that they cannot be sur-
prised.

— Gertrude Stein, American-French
writer, *Everybody's Autobiography*, 1937

WHEN MEDIUM-HIGH
SERIOUSNESS
COMPLETELY
REPLACES A
SENSE OF HUMOUR

About the only thing good you can say about old age is, it's better than being dead!
— Stephen Leacock, Canadian humourist, "This Business of Growing Old," *Reader's Digest*, March 1940

NO FURTHER
COMMENT
REQUIRED

They say wisdom comes as you age—
Now I'm in a real jam—
at sixty I should be a sage—

look what a fool I am!
— S. Minanel, American editor and poet,
"Maybe at Eighty?"

ON BEING NOT ALL THAT
OLD YET, REALLY

We forget all too soon the things
we thought we could never forget.
— Joan Didion, novelist, journalist

ON TAKING THE
LONGER VIEW

Next to the very young, I suppose
the very old are the most selfish.
— William Makepeace Thackeray,
English novelist, *The Virginians*, 1859

LIFE FOREVER FOLLOWS ART

It's never too late—in fiction or

life—to revise.
— Nancy Thayer, American writer

OR, FOR SOME OF US AT LEAST,
THE SECOND-MOST
UNEXPECTED THING?

Old age is the most unexpected of
all the things that happen to a man.
— Leon Trotsky, Russian revolutionary,
Diary in Exile, 1935

THOUGHTS ON
CREPUSCULARITY

That vague, crepuscular time, the
time of regrets that resemble
hopes, of hopes that resemble regrets, when youth has passed, but

old age has not yet arrived.

— Ivan Sergeyevich Turgenev,
Russian novelist,
Fathers and Sons, 1862

A CERTAINE CATTINESSE
IN THE SIXTEENTH CENTURY

The years that a woman subtracts
from her age are not lost. They are
added to another woman's.

— Diane de Poitiers,
16th century

REHEARSED AGAIN IN
THE TWENTIETH

Another woman's aging is thought
to be a victory for oneself, like win-
ning a race; one's own aging makes

one feel inferior.

— Paula Caplan, Canadian psychologist,
Between Women: Lowering the Barriers,
1981

AND THAT'S THE
RUB OF IT

No one is so old that he cannot live
yet another year, nor so young that
he cannot die today.

— Fernando de Rojas,
Spanish writer,
La Celestina

AND NO DOUBT THE
BESTEST IN THE WESTEST

Is not old wine wholesomest, old
pippins toothsomest, old wood
burn brightest, old linen wash

whitest? Old soldiers, sweethearts,
are surest, and old lovers are
soundest.
— John Webster, English dramatist,
Westward Hoe, 1607

EVEN WINDY
PLATITUDES
EVENTUALLY BLOW
THEMSELVES OUT

On such journeys, time is our ally,
not our enemy. We can grow wise.
As the arteries harden, the spirit
can lighten. As the legs fail, the soul
can take wing. Things do add up.
Life does have shape and maybe
even purpose.
— Sylvia Fraser, Canadian author,
My Father's House, 1987

STILL SOMEWHAT
CONFUSED
ON THE SUBJECT

Death happens and that's that. Age is worse in a way.

— Betty Friedan, American writer

WHAT AGE
DOESN'T DO

A woman may develop wrinkles and cellulite, lose her waistline, her bustline, her ability to bear a child, even her sense of humour, but none of that implies a loss of sexuality, her femininity . . .

— Barbara Gordon, American TV
producer and writer

POSSIBLY ANOTHER WAY
OF PUTTING IT

I have everything now I had twenty
years ago—except now it's lower.

— Gypsy Rose Lee,
American entertainer, writer

EVIDENCE THAT AGE, TO
SOME EXTENT, DOESN'T
NECESSARILY PROTECT
ONE FROM FATUITY

Age does not protect you from
love. But love, to some extent, pro-
tects you from age.

— Jeanne Moreau,
French actress

OR CERTAIN DARK TRUTHS,
FOR THAT MATTER

Old age is an island surrounded by death.

> — Judan Motalvo,
> Spanish writer,
> *On Beauty*

IN THOSE BLEAK AND
ANCIENT DAYS

Old age is the harbour of all ills.

> — Bion of Borysthenes,
> Greek philosopher, 4th century BC.

ONLY ONE WAY TO
ANSWER THIS ONE?

At seventy-four I look better than seventy-three. If you can make it through seventy-four years, can it be that things shape up?

— Ruth Gordon,
American actress, writer

INVOCATION FOR THE AGES

Grow old along with me!
The best is yet to be,
The last of life, for which the first
was made.
Our times are in his hand.

— Robert Browning, English poet,
Rabbi Ben Ezra, 1864

HOW ONE OUGHT TO
MEASURE ONE'S DAYS

A man is as old as his arteries.

— Thomas Sydenham,
English philosopher

TELL THAT TO MY FAILING
EYESIGHT, MY ACHING SCIATICA

To be old is a cultural concept.
— Merrily Weisbord, *Our Future Selves*

WHICH IS TO SAY, WE'RE ALL
AFRAID OF SOMETHING

Many men seem to be much more
fearful of death, while women are
more fearful of aging.
— Maggie Scarf, American writer,
Unfinished Business, 1980

OH, TO KNOW WHAT THOSE
CERTAIN OCCASIONS AND
POSSIBILITIES WERE!

I think I don't regret a single
'excess' of my responsive youth—I
only regret, in my chilled age,

certain occasions and possibilities I
didn't embrace.
— Henry James, American novelist

IS IT THE CART,
THE HORSE
OR THE ASSUMPTION
THAT COMES FIRST?
Of all the self-fulfilling prophesies
in our culture, the assumption that
aging means decline and poor
health is probably the deadliest.
— Marilyn Ferguson, American writer,
The Aquarian Conspiracy, 1980

VIEW FROM THE OTHER
SIDE OF
THE HILL
There's no such thing as old age;

there is only sorrow.
— Edith Wharton, American writer
A Backward Glance, 1934

PATHS LESS

TRAVELLED BY

I grow old ever learning many things.
— Solon, Athenian lawgiver,
poet, Fragment 22

METAPHORICAL ROADS

CONTINUE TO DIVERGE

*For age is opportunity no less
Than youth itself.*
— Henry Wadsworth Longfellow,
American poet,
"Morituri Salutamus," 1875

ON VALOUR AND
ITS BETTER PART

Vigor is found in the man who has not yet grown old, and discretion in the man who is not too young.

— Onasander, Greek playwright,
The General

ON WHAT A
GIRL NEEDS

From birth to age eighteen, a girl needs good parents, from eighteen to thirty-five she needs good looks, from thirty-five to fifty-five she needs a good personality, and from fifty-five on she needs good cash.

— Sophie Tucker,
American singer

WHAT WE PRAY
FOR THOSE WE LOVE

But an old age serene and bright,
And lovely as a Lapland night
Shall lead thee to thy grave.
— William Wordsworth, English poet,
To a Young Lady, 1807

YOUTH'S ELIXIR
AVAILABLE TO
SELECT FEW

Judges don't age. Time decorates them.
— Enid Bagnold, English playwright,
writer, *The Chalk Garden,* 1953

NO DENYING
THOSE DARK
NIGHTS

Being over seventy is like being
engaged in a war. All our friends
are going or gone and we survive
amongst the dead and the dying as
on a battlefield.

— Muriel Spark, Scottish writer,
Memento Mori, 1959

MORE OF THAT ETERNAL
VERITY, PLEASE

The same old charitable lie
Repeated as the years scoot by
Perpetually makes a hit—
'You really haven't changed a bit!'

— Margaret Fishback,
American writer

TURNING THE WHEEL
OF THE
GENERATIONS

Little by little,
I am becoming
my mother's mother.

— Natasha Josephowitz, Professor of
Management, lecturer,
Is This Where I Was Going?

WHAT THERE IS
TO BE PREFERRED
IN IT ALL

Age in a virtuous person, of either
sex, carries in it an authority which
makes it preferable to all the pleasures of youth.

— Sir Richard Steele, Irish essayist,
The Spectator

THERE ARE TIMES
WHEN IT MIGHT BE
CONSIDERED A VICE

Being seventy is not a sin.
— Golda Meir, Israeli Prime Minister

OR WHILE YOU'RE TRYING TO
COME UP WITH SOMETHING
CUTE TO SAY ABOUT IT

Life is something that happens to
you while you're making other
plans.
— Margaret Millar, American novelist

ONLY TO RAISE THE QUESTION
HOW SOON DOES
THE PRESENT TURN
INTO THE PAST?

What a wonderful life I've had! I

only wish I'd realized it sooner.

— Colette, French novelist

**THESE ARE THE DAYS THAT
MUST HAPPEN TO YOU**
*Youth, large, lusty, loving—
youth full of grace, force,
fascination,
Do you know that Old Age may
come after you with equal
grace, force, fascination?*
— Walt Whitman, *Leaves of Grass*, 1855

**ONE FOR THE
BATHROOM MIRROR**
Old age is the verdict of life.
— Amelia Barr (Edith Huddleston),
English-American writer, *All the Days
of My Life*, 1913

A METAPHOR TO
CARRY IN
THE HEART

Having gleefully chased butterflies in our young days on our way to school, we thought it might be as well to chase them in our old age on the way to heaven.

— Elizabeth Cady Stanton,
American suffragist

NOT TO MENTION
GOING ON RATHER
FATUOUSLY WHENEVER
THE FIT TAKES ONE

I postpone death by living, by suffering, by error, by risking, by giving, by loving.

— Anaïs Nin, French writer

ON WHAT
LINGERS

*Their eyes mid many wrinkles,
    their eyes
Their ancient, glittering eyes, are
    gay.*

— William Butler Yeats, Irish poet,
    "Lapis Lazuli," *Last Poems*, 1936

ON WHAT
REMAINS

All your past except its beauty is
gone, and nothing is left but a
blessing.

— Marianne Williamson,
    American writer,
    A Return to Love

POSSIBLE

LAST WORDS

I'm not mad, I'm just old.

      — May Sarton, *As We Are Now*

IF THERE BE ONE THING

TO SUSTAIN US IN

THIS SUBLUNARY WORLD

The hardest years in life are between ten and seventy.

      — Helen Hayes, American actress

EVELYN STEINBERG &
MARILYN WILLIAMS

Evelyn Steinberg is a principal and Marilyn Williams is a teacher working for the North York Board of Education in Ontario, Canada. Neither would divulge their age.

It is the purpose of Little Red Books to gather the essential wisdom of great women and men into single volumes so that students of the Great might judge them in light of their own words and the words that others speak of them, to find where they will the spiritual and sporting models so earnestly sought after by the young, and so often forgotten by the old.

LITTLE RED BOOKS:
THE COMPLETE LIBRARY

The Little Black & White Book of Film Noir

The Little Blue Book of UFOs

The Little Green Book:
Quotations on the Environment

The Little Greenish-Brown Book of Slugs

The Little Grey Flannel Book:
Quotations on Men

The Little Pink Book:
Quotations on Women

Quotations for a Nation

Quotations from Chairman Ballard

Quotations from Chairman Cherry

Quotations from Chairman Lamport

Quotations from Chairman Zalm

Quotations on the Great One